Intermittent Fasting

The Ultimate Beginner's Guide To Intermittent Fasting 16/8 Eating Plan Diet For Men & Women - Meal Timing Weight Loss "Secret" To Feel Energized, Burn Belly Fat On Cruise Control

By Logan Thomas

For more great books, visit:

EffingoPublishing.com

Download another book for Free

We want to thank you for purchasing this book and offer you another book (just as long and valuable as this book), "Health & Fitness Mistakes You Don't Know You're Making," completely free.

Visit the link below to signup and receive it:

www.effingopublishing.com/gift

In this book, we will break down the most common health & fitness mistakes, you are probably committing right now, and will reveal how you can quickly get in the best shape of your life!

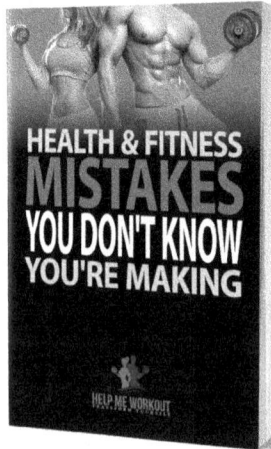

In addition to this valuable gift, you will also have an opportunity to get our new books for free, enter giveaways, and receive other useful emails from us. Again, visit the link to sign up:

www.effingopublishing.com/gift

TABLE OF CONTENTS

INTRODUCTION

This book is born from the idea of collecting in a single volume the necessary information of the intermittent fasting 16:8, an alternative approach to nutrition that in recent years has become very famous even in the world of show business.

This book does not want to replace the medical opinion, which is therefore preferable to consult before starting any diet type.

Also, before you get started, I recommend you joining our email newsletter to receive updates on any upcoming new book releases or promotions. You can sign-up for free, and as a bonus, you will receive a gift. Our *"Health &*

Fitness Mistakes You Don't Know You're Making" book! This book has been written to demystify, expose the top do's and don'ts and to finally equip you with the information you need to get in the best shape of your life. Due to the overwhelming amount of misinformation and lies told by magazines and self-proclaimed "gurus," it's becoming harder and harder to get reliable information to get in shape. As opposed to having to go through dozens of biased, unreliable, and untrustworthy sources to get your health & fitness information. Everything you need to help you has been broken down in this book for you to easily follow and to immediately get results to achieve your desired fitness goals in the shortest amount of time.

Once again, to join our free email newsletter and to receive a free copy of this valuable book, please visit the link and signup now: www.effingopublishing.com/gift.

According to the definition of the World Health Organization, health is "a state of complete physical, mental and social well-being and not merely the absence of illness or infirmity.

Maintaining health depends to a large extent on human nutrition.

We understand the difference between FOOD and NUTRITION.

FOOD is a voluntary choice, a choice we make of the food we want to eat.This is dictated by sight, taste, smell, or even a thought.

NUTRITION is the nutrient that has food that I decided to eat.

If I choose a pizza, from the moment it passes from the esophagus, the organism uses the nutrients necessary to it eliminating the waste.

So, the diet is voluntary while nutrition is involuntary, that I decide what to eat. Still, once ingested, I no longer have any power to determine whether or not to assimilate fat rather than the sugars contained in that food.

It is well known. Now reading the labels of the packaged products we buy should be a priority, but unfortunately, we are often deceived by advertising and the very appearance of food. Often, even in healthy products, sugars, preservatives, and trans fats are hidden, which are harmful to our bodies. It would be enough to turn the packaging of any product to find that the sugar appears among the first four ingredients. The ingredients written on the packaging are given in increasing order of quantity. Yogurts and biscuits, therefore, become dangerous foods for the line, but not only! Also, for the same metabolism. Imagine, for example, wanting to have breakfast with yogurt and biscuits with a little jam. We do not notice, but if both in the yogurt and the cookies are present sugars, our body will only produce insulin to lower the glycaemic peak occurred. Consequences? Tiredness, swelling, hunger just after an hour from the consumption of them. In detail, in which foods can harmful ingredients be found? First of all, as mentioned, in the biscuits also of well-known brands, yogurt, juice, bread box, muesli, cornflakes, bars, sauces like ketchup, but the list could go on indefinitely! How to fix it? Do conscious shopping, buy especially natural foods.

Why do we get fat?

The most common type of obesity is, however, what is defined as primitive or essential in which the accumulation of adipose tissue is the consequence of a positive energy balance. The body transforms the excess energy resulting from the imbalance between the too many calories introduced by diet and the few calories consumed in daily activities into fat, which is then stored in fat cells with resulting in increased body weight. In most cases, the cause of this energy imbalance is due to improper eating habits and reduced physical activity.

The countries most affected by obesity and overweight are the industrialized countries compared to the developing ones.The leading causes are to be attributed both to the increase in the consumption of very dense foods and high in simple sugars and saturated fats (which the industry proposes and advertises as "genuine and harmless"). Both to the increase in physical inactivity and laziness, that is the cause of what the French doctor Louis-Ferdinand Céline had called "epidemics of diseases from the full belly."

Slimming diets are generally based on a low-calorie regimen aimed at reducing calorie intake with foods, favoring foods that are less rich in calorie nutrients such as lipids and carbohydrates. There is a fundamental rule to follow if you are trying to lose weight or weight: if you want to lose weight, you have to eat fewer calories than you burn. If you're going to put pressure, you have to take more. This is true in quantitative but not qualitative terms: your body composition (percentage of muscles and fat to be understood) can be different in equal weight, and this depends on the quality of the food and the subdivision into macronutrients (proteins, carbohydrates, and lipids).

The role of the power supply is to provide the energy needed to meet the energy and plastic requirements of the "biological engine." For example, the dietary needs of the athlete or of those who systematically practice motor activity must take into account those that are the consumption during the training (and therefore also the daily habits of the individual) and during the competitions (food ration before or during the race).

According to Martin Berkhan, creator of the Lean Gains Protocol, during the period of our fasting, we will not be able to eat anything that adds calories to our body, but this does not mean that we cannot take anything. Berkhan comments that we can have coffee (preferably alone or with a tiny stream of milk), zero-calorie sweeteners, sugar-free chewing gum, or dietary soda (although I would be cautious with soft drinks called dietary).

Also, within this period, we can take infusions (there are countless flavors and aromas) that will make us less heavy to be drinking all the time water.

Why do diets fail?

When you start a slimming path, motivation is usually very high. One expects to lose weight quickly, continuously, and then be able to return to previous life rhythms. However, diets often require sacrifices in economic terms (food inspection and purchase), in time (food preparation) and personal (menu) that, in many cases, people are not willing to do for very long periods.

Many overweight people tend to confuse hunger with the desire to eat, have a low tolerance of hunger and cravings for food, love the feeling of satiety, are not aware of the amounts of food ingested. They console themselves with food, they feel hopeless when they get fat, they think the world is unfair because other people eat without getting fat, they stop their diet after the first period of weight loss.

From a practical point of view, when we deprive ourselves of food, perhaps because we are following a low-calorie regimen, our brain increases the sense of reward, increasing our desire to eat. That is not all, because this mechanism is manifested, especially with high-calorie products, such as chocolate ice cream or French fries. We will have experienced it on our skin: we will hardly want a dish of salad, but it is easier than a lovely carbonara.

An important fact to note is that our fat is not determined by genetics or at birth, you become fat when young. Excessive nutrition in childhood increases the "fat point" and will then imprint our growth. This thick point can remain dormant for mountains years and then wake up for various reasons (menopause, stress, hormonal alterations, etc.), giving the obesity of adult or late obesity. So, children need to eat properly to avoid carrying those extra pounds even in adulthood.

Diet and exercise: which is most important?

Remaining that the right thing to do would be to mix both aspects (exercise + proper nutrition), what science shows us that it is highly unlikely that weight loss comes only from exercise. Many studies say that weight loss is stimulated, especially by what enters our body rather than what we sweat. This is partly due to the way our bodies work: the majority of the energy we spend – about 60-80 percent– is what we need to survive, what we commonly call the basal metabolic rate. About 10 percent of our energy is spent on digesting food. So, activity, including formal physical exercise, can only represent 10-30 percent of energy expenditure.

Unfortunately, then some psychological aspects should not be underestimated. For example, sometimes, when we exercise and overcompensation mechanism triggers. In other words, we might be tempted to reward ourselves for a good workout with an extra plate. Or, exercise can make us feel hungrier, with a tendency to eat more. It is quite clear that each of these things can easily undo any weight loss benefit we might have had from the exercise. This does not mean that we should abandon training. As we know, exercise is excellent for the body and mind and offers us a wide range of health benefits.

The benefits of sports on body and mind

As we know, sports are indispensable to keep fit and live well. Sports help to lose weight and tone. It is also useful to the mind.

The most recent recommendations from the US and UK suggest regular periods of physical activity with moderate intensity. This type of movement, such as a sustained walk, is believed to be practicable for a much higher percentage of the population, as it can reasonably be inserted into everyday habits and requires less physical effort. Depending on the type and intensity, the movement improves different health and fitness factors. For example, a quiet walk at lunchtime, while not intense enough to improve circulation, can represent a healthy break from work, improve mood, and reduce stress, also contributing to weight control. For those who do not like scheduled exercise or fail to practice it, it may also be useful to avoid or reduce sedentary activities, such as watching television. To achieve maximum benefits for all parts of the body, however, specific strengthening and stretching exercises are also needed, particularly crucial for the elderly.

Sport makes you lose weight. Following a correct diet is not enough to lose weight and restore a satisfactory physical form. It is necessary to combine a healthy diet with constant physical exercise.

Especially in children, it reduces the risk of obesity. It improves cardiovascular activity, implementing the functioning of the heart and the consequent transport of blood and oxygenation of muscle and brain tissues.It is suitable for muscle tissues, strengthening them and making them more elastic and oxygenated, reduces blood pressure, and improves metabolism. Exercise is the best way to accelerate metabolism and increase energy consumption. The reasons are different. Regardless of the activity, you do: HIIT training, weight workout, cardio-training, or any other sport, through movement, consume many calories. But that's not all. The high-intensity training forms maximize the heartbeat; the body needs much more time to restore the heart rate to its resting values. It continues to burn more calories than it does, instead, if you practice endurance sports at moderate intensity. This phenomenon is called a post-combustion effect and is stimulated in particular by weight training and interval training during endurance training.

Regular physical activity can exert a beneficial effect on disorders and diseases affecting muscles and bones (such as osteoarthritis, back pain, and osteoporosis). Training exercises strengthen muscles, tendons, and ligaments and improve bone density. The data show that physical activity programs aimed at muscle strengthening help older people maintain balance, resulting in a reduction of possible falls.

Several specific studies have shown that physical activity can reduce clinical depression and can have the same effectiveness as traditional treatments, such as psychotherapy. Regular physical activity, over several years, can also reduce the risk of recurrence of depression.It is proven that movement improves the well-being of people who do not suffer from mental disorders. Numerous studies have documented an improvement in well-being, mood, emotions, and self-perception in terms of physical appearance, appreciation of one's body, and self-esteem.Also, both sporadic activity and training programs reduce anxiety, improve the reaction to stress, and the quality and duration of sleep.

It has also been shown that exercise improves various aspects of mental function, such as the ability to make decisions, to plan, and short-term memory.

Physical activity seems to be particularly healthy in older people because it can help to reduce the risk of dementia and the onset of Alzheimer's disease.

In general, sport changes the structure and function of the brain. Studies on guinea pigs and people have shown that physical activity generally increases the volume of the brain and can reduce the number and consequences of age problems in the grey and white matter of the brain. Sport also increases adult neurogenesis; that is, the formation of new neurons in an already mature brain.

What is intermittent fasting, and how does it work?

Today the food is available almost always, quickly and at a low cost. The temptation is still lurking. However, if our body is nourished continuously, it does not need to draw on its reserves. As a result, excess calories are converted into fat deposits, and our weight increases. During the intermittent fasting, the body is forced, for a specific time, to resort to its reserves. This is the advantage of intermittent fasting. Because one thing is sure: our organism does not need to eat continuously. Three main meals and, if necessary, two snacks are usually sufficient.

Intermittent fasting is a new way to lose weight fastly and easily. It is prevalent among athletes, and it is considered a good idea to lose weight and burn fats. Intermittent fasting is a strategy also applied in the field of fitness and bodybuilding, both in terms of the slimming phase and that of body recomposition. The supporters of intermittent fasting believe that by creating a precise time window in which they do not take food, can significantly affect the overall energy balance and also the metabolism of the various hormones. It seems that when you fast, you reach the so-called insulin calm (It should be remembered that insulin, the anabolic hormone par excellence, is responsible for lipid metabolism), stimulates the production of testosterone, and somatotropin (a hormone that increases hypertrophy and reduces fat deposits).

One of the inspiring principles of intermittent fasting is probably to be traced back to the origins of human nature: ancient hunters and farmers could pass even whole days without finding food, but they were able to find and use the energy they needed to continue looking for him. Based on this finding, various fasting methods have been tried and certified.

As well as being rooted in the prehistoric era where it was practiced for instinctive and environmental reasons, fasting was also widespread among various religions to enliven the soul and spirit towards purity and truth. Even different philosophers (Plato, Socrates, Pliny the Elder, and Plutarch, to name a few) have had direct experiences with fasting to stimulate intelligence and clarify ideas: Stimulating the release of catecholamines such as adrenaline and norepinephrine during the fasting hours improves attention and concentration.

Scientific studies prove that a restriction of calories promotes weight loss while maintaining lean mass. Intermittent fasting helps to ensure that your body does not use sugar as the first source of energy. Still, fats, also reducing the desire for sugars: when your body does not need sugar as the primary source of energy, you have a less hungry sense than when your sugar reserves drain out quickly.

One of the worst side effects of diet is that the body tends to burn both muscle and fat. It is interesting to note that some studies show that intermittent fasting can help maintain muscle and maximizing body fat loss. In a study, intermittent calorie restriction caused weight loss, such as continuous calorie restriction, but with a much smaller reduction in muscle mass.

The intermittent fasting 16:8 and has been tested on obese individuals, in particular, 23 with an average age of 45 years and an average body mass index of 35 (taking into account that 30 is the threshold beyond which for the WHO we speak of obesity).

The study continued for 12 weeks, during which the volunteers only ate what they wanted from 10 to 18. Still, they had to remain completely fasting for the remaining 16 hours, being able to drink only water or drinks without calories. Researchers found that obese people who had followed the 16:8 intermittent diet consumed fewer calories, lost weight, and had improvements in blood pressure.

After about 12 hours of fasting (the time varies slightly from person to person), the body will have exhausted the glucose present in the blood and that preserved as glycogen in the liver and muscles. With a shortage of energy, our body will be obliged to burn fat to meet all its needs

It is also a type of diet that supports the elimination of toxins and various harmful substances that can generally accumulate in multiple meals, allowing more natural purification of the organism.

Working with human and mouse immune cells, researchers have shown that intermittent fasting reduces the release of pro-inflammatory cells called "monocytes" into the bloodstream. Further investigations have revealed that during periods of fasting, these cells become "dormant" and are less inflammatory than the monocytes found in those who have eaten instead. "Monocytes are highly inflammatory immune cells that can cause severe tissue damage and there has been an increase in their circulation in the blood due to the dietary habits that humans have acquired in recent centuries .. Fasting could be the answer to the problem.

Intermittent fasting is not a real diet but a food program that consists of eating more or less alternately in a day\week.

To sum up, the critical principle of intermittent fasting is to create a space, a period of fasting that has a duration that can affect the total calories ingested and, therefore, the hormonal metabolism.

The different type of intermittent fasting

There are a lot of types of intermittent fasting:

-5:2, two days a week You have to reduce your intake of calories until 500\600 calories maximum. During these two days must not be consecutive and for the rest of the days, you can eat what you want.

-6:1, it is similar to 5:2, but in this case, you have to reduce your intake of calories only for one day. It works like this: For breakfast, you can eat two nuts, yogurt, kefir, and tea. At lunch, some broth and vegetables cooked to finish with a light dinner of non-amidaceous vegetables. For the rest of the week, you follow a Mediterranean diet, mainly vegetables.

-Lean day: you have to choose one day a week of calorie restriction in which to consume only vegetables, low fats (nuts, extra virgin olive oil), probiotic foods and fibers

-Eat stop eat, you are fasting for 24 hours for one or two days a week alternately, and during the rest of the days, you can eat. During the fasting hours water and some vegetables are allowed, while in the 48 hours of re-feeding, it would be advisable to follow a balanced diet, balanced and preferably with a low glycaemic load;

-Intermittent fasting of the warrior diet: your day must be organized on 20 hours of fasting (during which are allowed little fruit and raw vegetables) and then 4 hours, which must coincide with dinner, where you can eat to satiety

-16:8, it is also called "lean gains," this plan divides a day into two parts: 8 hours where you can eat and 16 hours of fasting.

-Method 14:10 It is similar to process 16: 8 but includes fasting for 14 hours and consumption for 10. It's a bit easier to perform, but it can be less effective when it comes to losing weight. Since fasting time is short and, more or less, follows people's dietary patterns, it can be challenging to lose weight with this type of diet.

-Fat loss Forever, an exciting fusion of the protocols mentioned above, it previews an alternation of the methods in several days of the week, joined to a precise workout to maximize the results, a sort of body recomposition-oriented program.

11 false myths on intermittent fasting and the frequency of eating

1) <u>Skipping breakfast makes you fat</u>

Although several observational studies have found statistical links between skipping breakfast and overweight/obesity, this can be explained by the fact that those who skip breakfast may already be departing a person who has no food awareness. This topic was recently addressed in a randomized controlled test. This study was published in 2014 and compared to those who had breakfast with those who jumped in a group of 283 overweight and obese adults. After a 16-week study period, there was no difference in weight between the two groups.

2) Meals often trigger and speed up metabolism

Many people believe that consuming more meals during the day leads to an increase in metabolic rate so that your body burns more total calories. Taking six meals of 500 calories has the same effect as eating 3 meals of 1000 calories. Given an average heat effect of 10%, it is 300 calories in both cases.

This is supported by numerous nutrition studies in humans, which show that an increase or decrease in the frequency of meals does not affect the total amount of calories burned.

3) *Eating frequently helps reduce hunger*

Some people believe that eating and snacking helps reduce excessive hunger and keep it under control. Although some studies suggest that more frequent meals lead to a reduction in appetite, other studies have not found significant effects, and others have even shown increased levels of hunger. In any case, no evidence snacking or eating more often reduces appetite in all.

4) *Making smaller meals helps you lose weight*Frequent meals do not boost metabolism (increase in calories burned).

They also appear not to reduce the feeling of hunger (reduction in calories introduced).This argument is supported by science. Most studies show that the frequency of meals does not affect weight loss.

For example, a study of 16 obese men and women found no difference in weight, weight loss or appetite compared to 3 and 6 meals per day.

5) *The brain needs a constant supply of glucose*

Some people believe that if you don't eat carbohydrates every five hours, your brain won't be more efficient.

This concept is based on the idea that the brain can only use glucose (blood sugars) as fuel.

In any case, what is often overlooked is that the body can quickly produce the glucose it needs through a process called glucogenesis. Even in a long period of fasting, deficiency, or in a diet with very low carbohydrate content, the body can produce ketones and nourish the brain with fats introduced into the diet. During prolonged fasting, the brain can easily sustain itself using the ketones of the body and the glucose obtained from proteins and fats.

6) *Eating often and snacking is right for your health*

It is simply unnatural for the body to be always in a state of nutrition.

During evolution, we have had to cope with periods of famine from time to time.

There is evidence that short-term fasting induces a cellular repair process called autophagy, in which cells use old and no longer functional proteins to extract energy. For example, a study found that combined with high-calorie intake, a diet with more frequent meals causes an increase in fat in the liver, indicating that snacks can increase the chances of fatty liver.

7) *The body can use a certain amount of protein per meal*

Some say we can only digest 30 grams of protein per meal and that we should eat every 2-3 hours to maximize muscle growth.

This concept is not scientifically supported.

Studies show no difference in muscle mass if you eat protein frequently.

8) *Fasting leads the body in "scarcity mode."*

A prevalent argument against intermittent fasting is that it can bring the body into a state of "scarcity and hunger."

According to these beliefs, not eating causes your body "to think "to be in famine, so it blocks your metabolism and starts burning less fat.

Long-term weight loss can indeed reduce the number of calories you burn. This is the true "scarcity mode" (the technical term is adaptive thermogenesis). A study showed that alternating days of fasting for 22 days did not slow the metabolism, but the participants lost 4% of the fat mass, which is impressive for such a short period.

9)*Intermittent fasting makes you lose muscles*Some believe that by starvation, our body begins to burn muscles and use them to get energy.

This indeed happens with diet in general, but there is no evidence that it happens more with intermittent fasting than with other methods. Some studies suggest that intermittent fasting is great for maintaining muscle mass.

In one study, the restriction of calories at intervals resulted in a similar amount of calorie loss as with a continuous calorie restriction, but less reduction in muscle mass. The intermittent fasting is also popular among bodybuilders, who have discovered that it is an effective way to maintain muscles with a low percentage of body fat.

10) *Intermittent fasting is harmful to your health*

Some believe that fasting can be detrimental, but nothing is further from the truth.

Numerous studies show that intermittent fasting and calorie restriction at intervals can have incredible health benefits, but we'll talk about this later.

11) *Intermittent fasting makes you eat more in periods of non-fasting*

Some argue that intermittent fasting does not

make you lose weight because it leads you to eat more in the interval where you eat.

This is partly true. After a fast, people automatically tend to eat a little more than when they have not been fasting. This is partially true. After a quick, people automatically tend to eat a bit more than when they have not been fasting. Intermittent fasting reduces total food intake and boosts metabolism. It also lowers insulin levels, increasing norepinephrine, and stimulating growth hormone by 5-fold. Thanks to these factors, intermittent fasting makes you lose fat, not gain it.

Focus on 16\8 intermittent fasting

Throughout our lives, we have been told that skipping meals was not good for our health and that we had to serve five meals, almost religiously. And yet in recent years, the diet protocol based on intermittent fasting has become very fashionable, and more and more people are following it.

The "fasting" is the total or partial abstention of food and drinks for a specific time.

"intermittent" means that this fast is periodically interrupted and controlled; therefore: The intermittent fasting is a diet pattern (not a diet) that alternates periods of total or partial abstention of food and drinks with normal feeding periods, on a regular and controlled basis.

As already written earlier, 16\8 intermittent fasting consists of eating only for 8 hours a day and fasting during the rest of 16 hours. In this case, we have to consider that reducing the time to eating in a day; we will also reduce the meals. You should consider fasting during breakfast. Still, you can have lunch and dinner until eight in the evening, or You can also choose to eat from nine in the morning to five in the afternoon and have a healthy breakfast and an equally tasty lunch, with some snacks before the fasting period. Ideally, the fasting period should coincide, in part, with the hours we spend sleeping so that we can spend part of that time sleeping and not feel the call of hunger that in the first few days you may feel when you are not used to it.

But if for whatever reason those hours we spend to sleep are few, another tip is that part of that fast agrees with you, for example, with your working day to keep you busy and that time passes faster, and you do not want to eat so much. If you have a stressful job, fasting protocol might not be a good idea, as stress makes excellent friends with hunger and food, and we could end up committing some "atrocity" against our body.

You can decide according to your needs. The recommended foods are fruit, vegetables, lean protein, and whole grains, while refined sugars, spirits, and sausages should be avoided.

You can toggle doing it one day to 7 days a week.

It's essential to know that intermittent fasting doesn't prohibit any food, but you have to adopt it as a healthy lifestyle, so you can't eat only junk food every day.

Why 16 hours of fasting?

Various scientific studies show that generally, we tend to be hungry during the same times of the day, and this fact is due to the release of ghrelin from cells located in our stomach. All this is controlled by circadian rhythms dictated by the times in which we have our meals.

For this reason, we usually try to keep more or less the 16 regular hours to find the right compromise between reaping the benefits and not having to suffer stress and too much hunger.

Fasting, however, is a practice that should not be improvised: the risks of depriving the body of the required energies can typically have serious consequences. For this reason, it is good to agree with a doctor and eventually change your lifestyle. The body must be gradually readjusted to endure periods of abstinence from longer food. Otherwise, all the benefits of fasting will be lost.

One of the most significant difficulties that people encounter when they approach intermittent fasting for the first time is the fear of facing periods of hunger being often accustomed to eating every 2-3 hours. The question you repeatedly hear when you propose an approach like fasting is how do I stay 12-16 hours without eating?

It is good to distinguish, in fact, the limbic hunger and the somatic hunger (coming from the stomach). The first comes when we face the food or think about it, it can also take place on a full stomach and usually occurs when we are used to eating at a particular time. This type of hunger is easily adjustable according to habits. It is a fake "hunger" as although presenting after 2-3 hours from the meal; the body is still in a state of "fed," likely, it is still digesting and using macronutrients from the last meal. Intermittent fasting is easy to do. Many people say they feel better and have more energy while fasting.

Eating plan diet for men and women

Breakfast is usually based on liquids and can then be eaten again in the hours of fasting (in fact it is skipped): lunch around noon, you allow a snack in the middle of the afternoon and dinner around 19 or 20. Afternoons and evenings can be used to relax and feed. So, this is not an absolute rule, but there is a large degree of flexibility about needs. There are also many positive effects on sleep quality and body composition in the intake of carbohydrates in the evening hours, amply demonstrated by the scientific community.

It is still possible to personalize the times observing the fast of 16 hours.

You have to distinguish the time of fasting from the time when you are allowed to eat: in the former, any food that you add calories would make an effort, but you can take drinks without added sugars such as tea, herbal tea, water or coffee.

Now we can analyze an example of an intermittent fasting plan for men and women.

For men

-Breakfast: you can drink a cup of coffee or tea without sugar;

-Lunch: a bowl of pasta\rice\barley\spelt (100grams) with vegetables, adding a spoon of olive oil and one fruit.

-Snack: 15 grams of nuts, 1 fruit, 70 grams of rice\mays cakes, tea or coffee without sugar.

-Dinner: Fish\meat (100grams, it's preferred white meat), cooked without fats. Then you can eat a plate of vegetables seasoned with a spoon of olive oil.

Women

Breakfast: you can drink a cup of coffee or tea without sugar;

-Lunch: a bowl of pasta\rice\barley\spelt (80grams) with vegetables, adding a spoon of olive oil and one fruit.

-Snack: 15 grams of nuts, 1 fruit, 50 grams of rice\mays cakes, tea or coffee without sugar.

-Dinner: Fish\meat (100grams, it's preferred white meat), cooked without fats. Then you can eat a plate of vegetables seasoned with a spoon of olive oil.

Another example could be:

-Morning: a cup of green tea or coffee;

-Snack: fruit with lots of water (like watermelon)

-Lunch: a sandwich with tuna or baked fish or piadina with vegetables and yogurt without fats;

-Snack: a piece of dark chocolate

-Dinner: lentil soup and grilled vegetables or grilled chicken breast and wholemeal bread;

An excellent draining herbal tea by INRAN

The draining herbal teas are many and one more tasty than the other. Nowadays, there is often no time to drink a lot during the day, and consequently, water retention is an increasingly common problem. The purpose of the draining herbal tea is precisely to promote the purification of the organism, even in the face of a quantity of water ingested less than necessary. Water retention has both aesthetic and health consequences. The skin is visually less fresh, is drier, cracked. Herbal teas usually consist of more substances, mainly because not all of them have a good taste or smell. Herbs for herbal teas are divided into three groups according to their function in the herbal tea: the constituent herbs are those that have the desired beneficial principle and have the main action; those adjuvants accompany the primary desired purpose of the other parallels; the corrective herbs serve instead to give the herbal tea a taste and a pleasant smell to the palate and the sense of smell.One of the plants best known for its draining action (even the sap is drunk for this purpose) is the birch, combining it with other draining substances such as the gramigna, the rod of gold, and the root of ononid we will have a tea with an intense draining effect.

The draining herbal teas have numerous beneficial effects, act positively on the lymphatic system and kidneys, prevent kidney stones, and the diseases mentioned above. In combination with drugs with a diuretic action, the draining tea can also act by facilitating the disposal of excessive lipid accumulation, helping the body against the edema of the legs, promoting the circulation, and disappearance of cellulite (for example, the red vine and the

Asian Centella). In the infection of the urinary tract, on the other hand, it is recommended to combine it with the bear grape and chamomile. It is clear that draining tea is not enough, but you need to lead the right lifestyle and containing, for example, the consumption of sodium. The herbal teas with draining properties are many. Of all tastes, everyone can then find his favorite consuming tea and also wanting to create original mixes; it is recommended, however, not to mix more than four sources. The draining drugs are the asparagus, the birch, the cherry, the horsetail, the ash, the gramigna, the corn, the ortosifon, the spiny ononide, the nettle, the saddle, the parsley, the dandelion, and the gold rod. If you buy these substances in herbal medicine, you will have the guarantee of a high concentration of the product. On the contrary, in supermarkets, it is easy to find herbal teas with more substances, many of which, however, are only mentioned for commercial purposes, given the small quantity present in the tea.

For maximum effect, the herbal tea should remain in infusion for thirty minutes and closing the cup (or pot) with the lid so that the volatile substances are not dispersing.

Here is a list of foods that you may want to eat:

- **Fruits:** Apples, berries, oranges, peaches, pears, grapefruit;

- **Veggies:** Broccoli (Broccoli are particularly rich in glucosinolates and isothiocyanates. Various studies have shown their antitumor action, especially for breast, colon and prostate cancer), cauliflower, cucumbers, leafy greens, tomatoes, zucchini, spinach, asparagus (contains glutathione, which can help purify the body. It is the most powerful and essential antioxidant produced by the body. It combats aging through two main ways: the intestine and the circulatory system. It protects the cells, tissues, and organs of the body, keeping it young.)

- **Whole grains:** Quinoa (Quinoa does not contain gluten and has very particular nutritional properties. The high biological value of its nutrients makes precious quinoa food. For the same weight, quinoa is among the grains - cereals or pseudocereals- with the most top content of vegetable proteins: quinoa proteins are bioavailable due to the presence of the significant essential amino acids, those necessary for the human body but only available through food. Contains proper amounts of linoleic acid, able to counteract and prevent damage due to a diet particularly rich in fats that damage the walls of the blood vessels, therefore useful against cardiovascular diseases, overweight, diabetes.), rice, oats, barley (It has anti-inflammatory properties, particularly in the bladder and intestine.

Being quite rich in fibers, it helps regulate intestinal function and is particularly useful in case of constipation), buckwheat;

- **Healthy fats:** Olive oil, avocados (also contains significant amounts of fiber and monounsaturated fats, beneficial in countering diabetes, and defending the heart. The avocado balances very quickly the level of "bad" cholesterol (LDL cholesterol) in the blood, thanks to its vegetable fats that reduce the time of residence of blood cholesterol: this benefits the whole cardiovascular system, especially concerning the balance of blood pressure. An inexhaustible source of vitamins: A (useful for sight), B1 (antineurotic), B2 (for growth and well-being), and also D, E, K,

H, PP. Its consumption is particularly suitable for children and for those who follow a vegetarian diet. It has aromatic, digestive properties and helps to fight dysentery, being an excellent astringent) and coconut oil (be an essential ally for those who want to lose weight: a 2009 study showed that consumption in women of 30ml (3 tablespoons) coconut oil per day for 12 weeks not only does not cause weight gain but also causes a reduction in abdominal or visceral fat, a hazardous and challenging type of fat to lose, which contributes to more significant heart problems);

- **Protein:** Meat, poultry, fish, legumes, eggs (Eggs are an essential source of protein and micronutrients, help regulate the intake of fats and carbohydrates, and according to many doctors contribute to the health of eyes, heart, blood vessels. Also, they contain vitamin A, riboflavin, folic acid (and therefore are essential in pregnancy), vitamins B6 and 12, choline, iron, calcium, phosphorus, and potassium. In particular, the yolk contains lecithin, which promotes the transport of cholesterol from the arteries to the liver, boosting the action of cholesterol "good"), nuts (Consuming daily a small ration of dried fruits such as peanuts, almonds, walnuts, hazelnuts, pine nuts, pistachios or cashews can be very useful because they are a source of essential nutrients for the daily diet. The high concentrations of protein (up to 20%), minerals, fatty acids, and amino acids make them irreplaceable. The regular consumption should be about 10 gr for those on a diet and about 20 g for those who are not on a diet), seeds like flax seeds (rich in Omega 3, Omega 6, and Omega 9; they also contain excellent antioxidants and fiber. It is recommended to take flax seeds after grinding them and let macerate in a liquid, to enjoy the benefits of this vegetable gel fully. They are useful to keep the colon healthy, reduce the risk of stroke and stroke and an anti-inflammatory).

Pumpkin seeds (an excellent source of magnesium, digestible vegetable proteins, B vitamins, Omega-3, zinc, and iron; are ideal for men as they protect from disorders attached to the prostate. They are also valuable to keep your mood high on difficult days and ensure a good sleep. Excellent for those who do diets, they are eaten raw, in smoothies, in vegetarian rolls, but also as a base sauce for pasta or ravioli. They are a good source of protein, thanks to tryptophan, a precursor amino acid of serotonin).

Fresh Fruit: Does it fatten?

Fresh fruit is low energy but highly nutritious food category, which means it is low in calories but rich in valuable nutrients such as vitamins, minerals, and fiber.

Consider the apple contains a lot of water. So, let's start well. If we then add fiber, low calories, and various proteins, such as pectin that stimulates intestinal peristalsis, we have found a new friend that will help us achieve the goal. We also remember the content of vitamins and antioxidants.

Blackberries are spontaneous fruits that are born and grow on the brambles, known for their thorns. They contain plenty of water and a few calories, which makes them great for losing weight. They also counteract constipation and exhaustion, promote diuresis, repair damage to the blood vessel walls, and delay the appearance of neurodegenerative diseases such as Parkinson's.

The autumn fruit to make a load of vitamins

Autumn, we know, is the bearer of the first ills. Rain and wind begin to knock at the doors, and getting sick is easy. There is, however, a way to help the body fight influence through nutrition. In particular, fruit and vegetables can help to strengthen the immune system, which is why I pay particular attention in my article to autumn fruit.

-Oranges, rich in vitamin" contribute to promote heart health, prevent tumors and kidney stones, anemia since they help to increase the absorption of iron, are a panacea for the skin and, strengthen the immune system. Rich in fibers. And tasty are classified as the favorite autumn fruit.

–Persimmons are very sugary and therefore have an energy function, purifying the body and are rich in antioxidants. Its pulp is used to create beauty masks

- Mandarin is a sweet fruit and is rich in vitamin c, fibers, and carotene. The tangerine peel is rich in lemonade, an antioxidant substance. Also, from the skin is obtained the essential oil of Mandarin, used, for example, against cellulite. As for nutrients, Mandarin is very rich in vitamin C but also contains B vitamins, vitamin A, vitamin P, Folic acid, and various minerals, including magnesium, potassium, calcium, and iron. Mandarin also contains bromine, a substance that promotes sleep and relaxation. It is easily digestible and, being rich in fibers, helps the smooth functioning of the intestine. It is a useful ally in the prevention of cooling diseases and helps protect capillaries and bones.

–Apples are composed mainly of fibers and mineral salts, are the dietary fruit for excellence, and have a draining effect. Does one apple a day take the doctor away? Absolutely

The apple is considered a natural medicine, a remedy for many problems. First, it must be said that this fruit contains very few proteins, and fats are almost absent (100 grams of apple corresponds to about 40 calories, 10 grams of sugar and large amounts of potassium, vitamin B, citric acid, and malic acid). Vitamin B1 is also present in it, which fights the loss of appetite, tiredness, and nervousness, and B2, which facilitates digestion, protects the mucous membranes of the mouth and intestine and strengthens hair and nails.

Eating legumes helps you lose weight.

Legumes help reduce the waistline. This is confirmed by recent studies conducted by the University of Otago (New Zealand) and recently published in the Journal of the American College of Nutrition. There are many beneficial effects that beans, peas, beans, chickpeas, keep in their pods.

Based on the slimming effect of legumes is their ability to increase the sense of satiety — all credit for the fibers. Even if these substances are not very important from the energy supplied (only 2 calories per gram) to include them in the daily diet is right for health, improves bowel function, and promotes the feeling of having a full stomach.

Legumes can be brought to the table as an alternative to meat, as it is an excellent source of protein. Unfortunately, however, they are deficient in some amino acids that are more present in other foods of vegetable origin, such as wheat, rice, and corn; for this reason, it is often said that the combinations of legumes and cereals (such as, for example, pasta, and beans, rice, and peas, or even pasta and chickpeas) are unique dishes perfect: they combine the amino acids of the first with those of the second, creating a mixture of protein of excellent quality.

Like all foods, if taken in excessive quantities, legumes can contribute to overweight. This is especially true when taken in the form of flour, in the mixed dough for bread or pasta, or as other derivatives such as tofu. Pulses in broth are more rarely taken in excess, which structures low-calorie and very satiating recipes.

Why is it better to prefer whole grains?

The nutrients contained in whole foods help our body to perform essential functions, bringing many benefits to our body. First of all, thanks to the fibers, they improve the digestion and the proper functioning of the intestinal tract. The vitamins and antioxidants help the immune defenses and slow the process related to cellular aging; starches under fiber control have less impact on glycemia and insulin, thus helping in the management of all those conditions associated with diabetes or otherwise to an altered response to carbohydrates. Regular consumption of whole-grain foods is generally essential for all in preventing certain types of diseases such as diabetes, constipation, and various gastrointestinal disorders.

The word integral tends to associate it with the idea of lean, but its true meaning is the exact opposite, which is rich, complete. Wheat, like all other cereals, deteriorates quickly when exposed to light and air. Thus, to increase the shelf-life of the food, it was thought to mechanically remove the most viable and oxidizable parts of the grain: the shell and the germ. The germ is usually the first to be eliminated because it is rich in fats that accelerate the process of rancidity. The bran, on the other hand, is separated for its taste a little too pungent, but in reality, it is the part that contains more fibers, minerals, and vitamins.

Not to mention the bleaching, a process that releases into the grinder's chemical residues harmful to health.

Cereals are whole grains, therefore, if and only if they have not undergone refining processes. And flour is only full when it contains both germ and bran. The insoluble fiber is beneficial in countering the high levels of cholesterol, as it can significantly reduce the absorption of cholesterol resulting from the diet at the intestinal level.

Why drinking green tea?

The human health benefits that can result from consuming green tea are many. This drink has already been and still is the subject of various studies, the aim of which is to know more and more about its possible curative role.

The leaves sprouts and young leaves of green tea contain the highest percentage of antioxidant principles found in nature, useful to counteract the formation of free radicals, responsible for cellular aging. The polyphenols present are anti-radical, even more potent than vitamin C and E.

Among the active substances that give the plant antimutagenic and anticancer properties, the most important is called epigallocatechin gallate (EGCG) because it inhibits the growth and proliferation of cancer cells. Another interesting property ascribed to green tea is slimming; due to methylxanthines (caffeine, theobromine, theophylline) with an effect on metabolism. They have hypoglycaemic action because they reduce the absorption of sugars, and lipolytic, as they promote the elimination of fats from adipocytes, by enzymatic stimulation. These substances, therefore, promote weight loss by facilitating the mobilization of fat localized in the fatty tissue and its removal for energy purposes.

This detoxifying action is effected through the diuresis: favoring as we have said the elimination of fats and sugars through the drainage of liquids, the intake of the plant is indicated in case of water retention, cellulitis and urinary tract infections such as cystitis. There's been a study published in the American Journal of Clinical Nutrition that says that one cup of green tea a day increases bone density in menopausal women for the powerful remineralizing action, which promotes the metabolism of bones and tissues. Also, the high percentage of fluorine allows the mineralization of the skeleton and tooth enamel (anti-caries).

Green tea accelerates the metabolism of fats and sugars, facilitating the decrease of body weight and promotes diuresis, being useful in case of water retention, cellulite, and urinary tract infections.

Green tea contains caffeine and high doses and can, therefore, cause anxiety and nervousness, nausea, and vomiting. For all these reasons, controlled consumption is essential. Do not take after 18 to avoid insomnia.

Foods rich in fiber, what are they, and why consume them? (By Inran website)

Fiber-rich foods can be an excellent ally of our well-being. Thanks to the protective and beneficial effect that they can exert on the organism. Many advantages can be achieved through a rich fiber diet. First of all, as repeatedly advertised also in commercial spots, the fibers have excellent effects on the intestinal and gastric tract, favoring the dragging of foods, with reduction of unwanted fermentations (and gas) and slowing the gastric transit time, with a decrease in the rate of absorption of the sugars taken together with the fiber. They also allow an increase in fecal mass, which facilitates elimination functions.

Among the other most important benefits, we can only recall the increase in the rate of satiety of foods, the reduction of cholesterol levels, and the reduction of carcinogenic and mutagenic substances within the intestinal tract. As if this were not sufficient to guide you towards greater consumption of fiber, we also point out the positive effects in terms of enrichment of the intestinal flora with useful microorganisms, and the strengthening of the wall of the entire digestive tract, with the prevention of diverticulosis.

For example, oat bran is not used for baking because it is gluten-free, but its nutritional values are often very high, comparable to those found in wheat.

This food contains very high fiber portions and a quantity of polyunsaturated fatty acids that occupy a prominent place, as well as an excellent supply of niacin and magnesium. As regards macro-nutrients, oat bran has a higher quantity than wheat bran, both lipid and protein, and there are also significant amounts of saturated fatty acids and monounsaturated fatty acids, while for polyunsaturated fatty acids are present in the same quantity in both portions of cereal.

The carbohydrates found in oat bran are in a much lower quantity than wheat bran.The usual consumption of oat bran promotes the absorption of fats and consequently decreases the blood cholesterol values.

As mentioned, it helps to promote intestinal transit by forming soft stools that are easy to sweat.

Due to the low amount of glycaemic index, take bran at least twice a week, counteract insulin formation after eating meals.

Vegetables for losing weight quickly.

In diet or maintenance, vegetables are an essential element. However, some vegetables help you lose weight faster, thanks to their draining or fat-burning properties. Find out which are the primary vegetables to lose weight to include in your daily menu.

1-LettuceGreen leafy vegetables and lettuce, in particular, are foods rich in vitamins and minerals, including magnesium. They contain fiber and are satiating. Lettuce has relaxing effects useful in case you suffer from anxiety, even more, if caused by slimming diets; contains 17 calories per 100 grams; The salad is provided with a particular molecule, glucochina, which makes this food particularly suitable for people with diabetes because it has a hypoglycaemic effect (lowers the level of glucose in the blood).

The lettuce extract has shown considerable control over the death of neurons due to its role in glucose (serum) deprivation (GSD). The research also mentioned that lettuce has the potential to be used as a remedy for neurodegenerative diseases. One of the main traditional uses of lettuce in the Hungarian medical system was as an inducer of sleep.

Isolating a particular chemical agent from the lettuce extract showed that when used on animal guinea pigs, it gave sedative effects. A decrease in heart rate and ventricular contractions was also observed.

2- OnionOnion is a great option to include in meals if you want to lose weight. It helps eliminate liquids, avoids constipation, and controls blood sugar levels. Useful for those suffering from water retention or to purify the kidneys. It is also rich in vitamins A, C, E, and B, but also in potassium, calcium, and sodium and is essential for its high content of Phyto-oestrogens and cannabinoids substances, which promote diuresis and thus the elimination of liquid stagnations.

3. Cucumbers; It is a vegetable with high water content and low in calories: the ideal for satiating and perfect for adding to salads but also as an ingredient for smoothies and extracts, as refreshing and diuretic. Tartaric acid in the pulp helps to block the transformation of carbohydrates into fats. The cellulose present promotes intestinal transit and eliminates toxins, as well as reducing cholesterol. It contains 15 calories per 100 grams.

4.Fennel

With only 9 calories per 100 grams, fennel is a crunchy and tasty snack, perfect for adding to the salad. They contain a lot of vitamin C and calcium and only 1% of sugars.

Vitamins become essential to protect the body, vitamin A keeps the skin healthy and regulates the functioning of the retina and vision; Vitamin B, is necessary for the proper functioning of the nervous system and the cardiovascular system, and vitamin C, strengthens the immune system and plays an effective antioxidant action. The excellent content of phytoestrogens makes fennel, an excellent natural balance of the levels of female hormones, which makes it particularly useful in stimulating milk production in women struggling with breastfeeding, to reduce disorders that precede the menstrual cycle and relieve the symptoms of menopause.

Eating fennel helps to reduce the glycaemic index of foods that are richer in sugar taken in the same meal. Having a high satiating power, then, this vegetable soothes the desire for both sweet and salty. It promotes purification and regularizes the intestine, deflating the stomach.

5- Zucchini

Zucchini are native to the American continent and are currently grown a little around the world. Their harvesting period coincides with the spring even if now, thanks to greenhouses and imports, they are present on the market all year round.

The presence of fiber favors the expulsion of excessive bad cholesterol. According to studies, pectin is the main type of fiber that has properties useful in reducing cholesterol. Consuming courgettes is, therefore, an excellent preventive method against the formation of dangerous plaques in the arteries.

Other studies confirm the anti-cholesterol LDL properties of the fiber present in the food. The soluble fiber can interfere with the absorption of bad cholesterol.

They are very low-calorie food, and that is why they are often based on their diet. The presence of fiber then increases the feeling of satiety and prevents the intake of other food in the short term.

It is a vegetable with a low glycemic index and is rich in water, the latter contributing to increase the sense of satiety. Studies suggest that the intake of fruit and vegetables and low-fat foods is useful for weight loss and maintenance

6- Spinach

Spinach contains iron, but the belief that it brings a large quantity to the organism is wrong. To facilitate the absorption of this mineral, it is advisable to consume spinach seasoned with lemon; vitamin C contained in citrus helps to absorb iron. Spinach is rich in vitamin A and folic acid. They are also rich in nitrate, a substance that has been the subject of recent research, as it appears to help increase muscle strength. They're useful in constipation.

Spinach not only makes us stronger but also faster and more responsive.

According to a recent study, spinach helps us to be more lucid and improves our reflexes. The merit is tyrosine, an amino acid that allows the brain to produce two fundamental neurotransmitters, such as dopamine and norepinephrine. Tyrosine is also present in other foods, such as beans, soya beans, and hazelnuts, as well as in some foods of animal origin.

7- The cauliflower

Cauliflowers are a source of antioxidants, which slow down the aging of cells. They are particularly rich in glucosinolates and isothiocyanates. Various studies have shown their antitumor action, especially for breast, colon, and prostate cancer. It is beneficial, therefore, to insert cauliflowers in your diet as a functional food rule.

The isothiocyanates, which contain an atom of sulfur, which derives the unpleasant smell that is released in the cooking, facilitate the elimination of the toxic substances and contribute to apoptosis, which is to the programmed death of the tumor cells. It contains carotenoids and flavonoids, two antioxidants that help decrease the risk of developing cardiovascular diseases. The former help to lower harmful cholesterol levels, thus reducing the risk of atherosclerosis and coronary heart disease. A study published in the American Journal of Clinical Nutrition suggests that a diet rich in flavonoids can promote the prevention of cardiovascular diseases. Cauliflower has few calories: 25 per 100 grams. So, you can eat many, without worrying. Being rich in fiber makes us feel full quickly. Besides, 92% of their weight is made up of water.

8- It contains potassium, phosphorus, magnesium and calcium, vitamin C, vitamin K, and, in smaller quantities, some B vitamins and vitamin E. Celery is composed of about 90% water; for this reason, it is diuretic and purifying. It contains lutein, a protective antioxidant against the brain. Celery is also a strong ally against hiatal hernia. Regular consumption of celery is useful in people with high blood pressure, as it can help to reduce blood pressure. Celery juice, always taken regularly, can help against rheumatism. It has very few calories and can, therefore, offer an excellent way to give flavor to sauces and sauces without almost increasing the calorie value.

8-Tomato

Thanks to its fiber adequately nourish the intestinal bacterial flora "good," promoting the correct balance of our intestine, which is essential to stay healthy and keep away from various diseases, not only cancers but also allergies, autoimmune diseases, and obesity. The tomato is then well equipped with bioactive molecules such as antioxidant polyphenols, precious against aging. It is also known for the content of an antioxidant, the lycopene that colors it red, and serves for the proper functioning of the immune system and the prevention of tumors. Vitamin C is better absorbed by eating raw tomatoes instead of lycopene if cooked: the temperature breaks the cell walls making it more usable. A valuable tip: pour on the cooked tomato a little extra virgin olive oil added raw to keep intact even the properties of the seasoning. Tomato sauce is a healthy food that can approach 'correct nutrition, even children. Each type of vegetable is rich in minerals, vitamins, and bioactive molecules.

Olive oil and benefits

Extra virgin olive oil is not just a seasoning, but a precious ally for health and beauty that should never be lacking on our table. Attention, however: although it is indispensable for a healthy diet, it is also true that it should not be abused or used in the wrong way.

Extra virgin olive oil contains healthy fats that help us keep the arteries clean. Also, it makes foods more digestible and also helps in case of constipation, because it facilitates the elimination of waste and the movement of intestinal villi".

Numerous studies confirm the virtues of olive oil: it reduces the risk of cardiovascular diseases, prevents the aging of the body, counteracts the onset of cancer, prevents asthma and arthritis because it reduces inflammation. This mix of substances beneficial to your body, acting in synergy, also has the effect of strengthening your immune system. The extra virgin olive oil is also indicated in periods of particular fatigue or stress, such as changes in season, a period of examination, or moments when an extra boost of energy is welcome: This is because of the vitamins and minerals it contains make it a strong tonic.

The calories introduced with extra virgin olive oil are not few, so we must make a smart and correct use for plots only the benefits.

The recommended amount is about one tablespoon per meal, which corresponds to about 15 grams. The dose may vary depending on age, gender, physical activity. Proper use means not only taking care of quantities but also their use in the preparation of dishes.

When raw, they assume all the qualities, not

only nutritional, but also organoleptic, such as aromas and perfume, but it is useless to hide the fact that we often use it for cooking, or even for frying.So let's see what happens with the heat to our oil brought to high temperatures, the olive oil loses its properties of monounsaturated fat.

Why eating white meat?

White meat has the advantages of noble proteins of animal origin, without the typical contraindications of red meat, fatter, longer to digest, and source of cholesterol.

For our diet, we will choose the various types of chicken, rabbit, turkey, to alternate with fish. We will exclude the duck and the goose, which, although they are poultry, due to their characteristics, are among the red meat.

White meat satiated without getting fat the ratio between the calories it provides (few), and the sense of satiety it gives is one of the highestIt also provides the best-assimilated proteins; in fact, the white meat has a sequence of amino acids that allows the best intestinal absorption.It contains tryptophan, a precursor of the neurotransmitters of well-being.It keeps your tissues firm even when you lose weight. Rich in noble proteins, the meat is precious for the protein replacement of the muscles; it is used to build them and to keep them firm during the weight loss.

It is good to renew tissues, and it contributes to the formation of enzymes and antibodies.It is well digestible, thanks to the low content of connective tissue, fat, and the reduced diameter of muscle fibers. This allows a quick action of gastric juices. It is easier to lose weight if you digest better.

Another advantage of white meat is that all the

fats it contains are concentrated in the skin and under the skin, where they are separated from the rest. Before cooking, remove the visible fat and remove the skin.

Is there any food that can be avoided to accelerate metabolism?

Yes.   In these products, we find dyes, preservatives, stabilizers, agglomerates, sweeteners, emulsifiers, acidity regulators, and so on, as well as some processing processes. In short, spreadable cheese is more harmful than a slice of camembert.

A slice of polyphosphate ham is more damaging than a piece of beef.

For example, food subjected to "sophistication": croquettes, soups, biscuits, spoon creams everything that has a list of ingredients that you do not fully understand, made of abbreviations, nomenclatures, and chemicals or all foods preserved in plastics and non-BPA films free, in cans without coating, in metal cans. They can contaminate the food with heavy metals, while BPA is an endocrine disrupter recently linked to obesity. Foods with sweeteners: Chemical and refined, although without calories or with lower glycaemic index, are even worse than sugar. Some studies have found that the consumption of artificial sweeteners is linked to an increased risk of metabolic diseases. True or yet to be verified, the more we consume sweeteners, the more we get used to an excessive and constant sweet taste. That recalls the desire of "real" sugar.

Another trend that companies exploit to win over the consumer are products with "fiber addition." Say that the products are rich in fiber, so healthy and dietetic compared to traditional products. But what kind of fiber is it? Also, here, the dashboard, in the luckiest cases, a percentage of inulin, pectin, gums: the result is a product full of fibers that can damage the intestinal villi and cause flatulence.

Even alcohol is also incredible and unsuspecting calorie bombs, even three hundred calories. It should also be remembered that alcohol (ethanol) provides 7 calories per gram, which are added to those brought in with food. It is therefore advisable to avoid spirits, which provide only empty calories 'without any health benefits, especially for those who are prone to overweight or already have an abundant waist. It is good practice to limit alcohol to occasional consumption only and in any case to compensate 'for excess calories with physical activity. Keep in mind that a woman of 50 kilos running at a speed of about 8 km now, in that hour, consumes about 400 kcal, the amount of calorie contained in 4 glasses of wine of 125 ml.

Recipes

Grilled chicken rags with zucchini and carrots

It is a dish of meat straightforward and fast to prepare. Chicken, being white meat and rich in protein, lends itself well to delicate and nutritious and balanced second courses, perfect for those who follow a healthy diet without sacrificing taste. Carrots and courgettes are perfectly combined with grilled rags in a light dish, definitely summer because fresh and colorful: a recipe that strikes for its simplicity.

Ingredients:

-chicken breast 100grams

-carrots 70grams

-zucchini 100grams

-Olive oil 1 spoon

Preparation method

1-First clean the chicken breast by removing the white filaments.

2-Heat a grill, and as soon as it is boiling, gently place the meat.

3-Cook for 5 minutes per side, turn off the heat, then cut the chicken into strips and let it cool.

4- Peel the carrots and cut into julienne and peel zucchini and cut into rounds;

5- In a non-stick frying pan, add the carrots, salt and cook for 2/3 minutes. Add the courgettes and cook over high heat for 5 minutes.

6-When the vegetables are cooked, add the chicken, sauté for a minute to make the meat taste, and add olive oil. Then serve immediately.

Risotto with pumpkin

Pumpkin risotto is a simple recipe, vegetarian, and gluten-free light so suitable for all people who follow special diets and diets, but also fast to prepare and exceptionally useful.

Ingredients:

-Brown rice 80grams

-Pumpkin 200grams

-Broth

-Olive oil 1 spoon

Preparation method

1- Clean the pumpkin, remove all the skin, and wash it thoroughly. Cut it into small cubes and put it in a pan. Cook the pumpkin for 5 minutes

2- Add the rice and let it toast for a few minutes.

3-At this point soak everything with a ladle of hot broth.

4-Continue cooking by adding the remaining boiling broth a little at a time. The risotto will be ready after about 15–20 minutes and should be very soft.

Lentil and spelt soup

This soup is excellent for the cold winter days in which you want to pamper yourself a little... healthy!

Lentils are a nutrient and dense product to add to your diet. The dried lentils consist of about 8% water, 26% protein, 63% total carbohydrates, and 42-47% starch. They are loaded with minerals and are a particularly good source of magnesium, calcium, potassium, zinc, and phosphorus. Their distinctive feature is that they are rich in essential amino acids – called lysine– than other grains do not have enough. However, it is also true that they lack another essential amino acid tryptophan. So, make sure you get sources from meat or other cereals.

Lentils help reduce blood cholesterol because they contain high levels of soluble fiber. Lowering cholesterol levels reduces the risk of heart disease and stroke by keeping the arteries clean.

Several studies have shown that eating fiber-rich foods such as lentils reduces the risk of heart disease. Lentils are also a great source of folic acid and magnesium, contributing significantly to the health of the heart. Folate lowers homocysteine levels, a severe risk factor for heart disease. Magnesium improves blood flow, oxygen, and nutrients throughout the body. Low magnesium levels have been directly associated with heart disease.

This recipe comes from the desire for something warm, especially in these days of snow. I have chosen to obtain a total weight of 80gr, but you can also reduce it to 60gr. The proportion is 1 to 1: a part of spelt and a part of lentils.

Spelt is a cereal belonging to the gramineous family, has gluten, and the flour can be used to produce bakery products: bread, pizza, etc....

Its nutritional value is 340 kcal per 100g and also contains mytonin, essential amino acid deficient in almost all other cereals.

Ingredients

-Spelt 40grams

-Lentils40grams

-Oil e.v.o: 5gr;

Preparation method

1. Soak the lentils in cold water for 12 h and then drain.

2. Pour the water back into the pot with the lentils and bring it to a boil;

3. Dip the spelt and cook for about 35 min or until it is semi-soft (the spelt

has its semi-hard consistency, it may seem raw);

4. Turn off and season with raw oil;

5. Consume!

Needed days to see a concrete weight loss

The days needed to see a changeset are 7 (minimum), but it is different from body to body; sometimes, our weight is influenced by stress, environment, and moisture.

There is no quantity of standard kilograms that those who experience this diet can lose; in fact, the positive effects must be sought in the reduction of the fat mass rather than in the variation of the figure displayed on balance.

The weight loss is proportional to the duration of the fast. It depends strictly on the calories taken in the second phase of the diet, although the physical activity is also contributing. The observed rapid initial weight loss is often water. Subsequently, it is estimated that you lose, on average, 500 g per day of fasting.

From the Harvard website: A randomized controlled study that followed 100 obese people for a year did not find that intermittent fasting is more effective than daily calorie restriction. [6] For the 6-month weight-loss phase, subjects were fasted alternately daily (alternating days of a meal of 25% of essential calories compared to 125% of necessary calories divided into three meals) or daily calorie restriction (75 % of crucial calories divided into three meals) following the American Heart Association guidelines. After 6 months, calorie levels were increased by 25% in both groups to maintain weight.

Benefits

As already mentioned, those who interpret human behaviour in the light of evolution argue that a style of nutrition, in which you alternate periods without food intake to moments when instead you eat freely, resemble conditions in which our species has evolved. It would, therefore, be a style that can best accommodate the physiological mechanisms developed during the evolutionary process.

Intermittent fasting allows you to eat normally after the temporary deprivation of food. The health benefit occurs at the cellular level. When the calorie intake is interrupted with food, then begins the so-called autophagy process: the "molecular waste" accumulated in our organism over time are collected and recycled. Japanese Yoshinori Ohsumi received the 2016 Nobel Prize for his work on this mechanism of self-cleaning and self-healing cells.

Although at the beginning, it may be challenging to adapt to change, in the medium and long term, the intermittent fasting reduces the impact of leptin (the hormone of satiety) on the body. When there is too much leptin circulating in the body, For example, when we eat regularly, the body develops resistance, and this means that it no longer reacts to this hormone and needs more and more food. Fasting lowers the leptin levels.

Intermittent fasting can produce the most significant benefits for those who are overweight. Still, people who have reached the plateau with their efforts to lose weight may find that intermittent fasting can help restart their metabolism and help with their progress.

It has been becoming increasingly evident for years that, by associating with a proper diet, periods of fasting relatively longer (than the classic nocturnal hours), it does not hurt, and, at least, could help establish "without traumas,." The calorie deficiency, which, besides being recognized as the first medicine for practically all metabolic diseases, is also the determining and indispensable factor for weight reduction. The latter, weight reduction, is just the other major factor for the prevention of diseases. A decrease of only 10% of one's body weight, at least initially, on obese subjects, or the maintenance of the shape weight in subjects with a BMI considered healthy and an acceptable fat mass (15% for men, 20-25% for women).

There is increasing scientific evidence that fasting and exercise are growth factors that activate the turnover and rejuvenation of the brain and muscle tissues.

These include BDNF growth factors and MRF muscle factors. They are the growth factors that signal the stem cells of the brain and the satellite muscle cells to transform respectively into new neurons and new muscle cells.Interestingly, the BDNF also expresses itself in the neuro-muscular system, where it protects neuro-motors from degradation.

Neuro-motor degradation is part of the process that explains age-related muscle atrophy.

Intermittent fasting changes hormonal balance, helping the body to use fat reserves. Specifically, it helps to:

-Enhance insulin sensitivity, primarily if you associate intermittent fasting and sport. If you have a low insulin level, it will be natural burning fats; When glucose is taken with food, it triggers a mechanism that leads to insulin release. This hormone, produced by beta cells in the pancreas, is responsible for the transport of glucose through GLUT transporters manages to enter the cell and be stored. Insulin has a hypoglycaemic effect by lowering the amount of blood glucose when it is high, especially after a glucidic meal, bringing it within a range of 80-120 mg/dl. When the glucose level rises above this range, insulin is released to return glucose to baseline levels.

Insulin exerts essential functions in lipid metabolism by favoring their conversion into fat as well as the absorption of glucose in the cells. In the presence of an insulin response, the body mainly uses carbohydrates as an energy substrate converting excess carbohydrates into lipids (excess glucose can be transported and stored inside adipocytes, thus facilitating fat accumulation). On the contrary, in its absence, the body uses mainly fatty acids.

-Your body will use fats like energy and increases the production of growth hormone, so your muscle mass will develop faster. GH release occurs due to the presence of stressors, including over-exercise, hypoglycemia, carbohydrate restriction, even fasting seems to lead to an increase in GH, especially during night hours. GH promotes protein synthesis, promoting the transport of amino acids, stimulates RNA synthesis, and the activity of ribosomes. GH also performs functions on lipid metabolism, promoting the reduction of the use of carbohydrates and an increase in lipid oxidation, promoting the mobilization of fats. Intermittent fasting (if set correctly) does not cause loss of muscle mass and would instead improve its maintenance. The GH spike that occurs during fasting hours could also inhibit the loss of muscle proteins.

-- Increase glucagon (lipolytic hormone): During periods of fasting, insulin tends to decrease. In this phase, however, another hormone has an almost opposite function to that of insulin, namely glucagon.

Glucagon is also produced in the pancreas (from alpha cells), but unlike insulin, its production increases during periods of fasting and decreases after a meal.

Glucagon performs its function in the liver leading to depletion of hepatic glycogen.

It has a hyperglycaemic and lipolytic effect because when the blood glucose tends to decrease (a fact that happens with fasting and with intense physical activity), the glucagon is stimulated to raise the glycemia and (using mainly fats) maintain constant glucose levels.

-Reduce triglycerides which simplifying, we can define forms of accumulation of excess energy introduced with diet and potential risk factor as well as for cardiovascular diseases also for insulin-presence and metabolic syndrome;

Insulin resistance, in medicine, means the low sensitivity of cells to the action of insulin, which can lead to type 2 diabetes mellitus. Causes can be hormonal (the most common), genetic, or pharmacological. Insulin resistance is closely associated with obesity. However, you may be resistant to insulin without being overweight or obese.

Modern research has shown that resistance to insulin can be combated by treatments, which help to reduce the amount of insulin the body is producing, or by making insulin dosages via under-skin punctures.

Reduced resistance to insulin can be achieved by using low-carbohydrate diets or ketogenic diets, including intermittent fasting.

-Substantial maintenance of HDL cholesterol levels, cholesterol "good," which according to some authors, would have a protective effect against cardiac and vascular pathologies; HDL is measured by analyzing its concentration in the blood serum. They are not all the same, and there are different types, which vary in shape, size, and chemical composition. The most effective in "cleansing" the arteries are logically the most active in the exchange of lipids with cells and other lipoproteins.

Each HDL is made up of 80-100 specific proteins, which make it able to convey even several hundred fat molecules at a time. The "supply" and "discharge to destination" of fats occur by the interaction of HDL with cells and other lipoproteins.

-Reduce the inflammatory state of the organism. This leads to a benefit against numerous chronic-degenerative diseases that develop right in the face of a chronic inflammatory condition;

-Improving the expression of genes because fasting seems to improve the way genes are expressed. These changes in function have been shown to protect against disease and promote longevity.

Fasting promotes autophagy and the best mitochondrial function

The autophagy is a physiological process of the body (comes from the Greek "eating themselves," also called "autolysis"), which takes place at the cellular level. It is present in all living organisms and consists of a mechanism that leads to the destruction of proteins or parts of the cell membrane. It is a significant event for the survival of the cell as it provides the necessary nutrients, when these are not available, through degeneration and recycling processes.Autophagy involves replacing the damaged and diseased parts of the cell with new components created by the organism itself to regenerate and rejuvenate". The body begins to sustain itself thanks to the use of some of its aging parts and, therefore, to replace it. Autophagy, in this way, expresses two benefits in one: it provides new energy to the body and at the same time, eliminates certain now dysfunctional parts.

-Reduce the oxidative stress, fasting decreases the accumulation of oxidative radicals in cells, thus reducing the oxidative damage of cellular proteins, lipids, and nucleic acids, associated with aging and disease. A state of oxidative stress results from the action of highly reactive unstable chemicals (the free radicals of oxygen and nitrogen, ROS and RNS), of non-proradicals pro-oxidants (such as hydrogen peroxide) and ionizing radiation. If the antioxidant defenses of the cell and the body are insufficient to maintain REDOX state in balance and the stress situation is prolonged, the excess of ROS and RNS can generate important changes that, in the long run, become irreversible.

-protect your brain fasting stimulates the production of a protein called brain-derived neurotrophic factor (BDNF), which stimulates the release of new brain cells and numerous other compounds that protect you from Parkinson and Alzheimer's.

-improve cognitive skills and memory;
-increase fatigue resistance and physical and mental energy;

-Fasting decreases the concentration of thyroid hormone T3, while the levels of thyroxine (T4) and free T4 remain the same or drop only slightly. Besides, the thyroid-stimulating hormone (TSH) does not increase.

Doesn't fasting slow your metabolism?The intermittent character of the fasting technique guarantees an always optimal level of our metabolism, which is a certain sense is still taken by surprise.

Another curious effect of intermittent fasting is an improvement in asthma symptoms:

Alternative daily calorie restriction improves clinical results and reduces markers of oxidative stress and inflammation in overweight adults with moderate asthma

Advice and advertisement

It is essential to fast at a time when you can rest without stress and drink plenty of water. Also, feeding must be programmed to make the best of our activities and never be a constraint on our commitments. Before doing an intermittent fasting test, talk to your doctor.

Another disadvantage is hunger during the fasting phase, especially during the first few weeks. You soon learn that hunger comes and goes, but you need a period of adjustment before your body gets used to the new regimen. After about three weeks, the morning hunger disappeared almost completely in my case, and

I had no problems even when I had to have lunch later than expected. However, in the morning, I tend to have slightly less energy than in the afternoon-evening.

The intermittent fasting, in all its forms, should be approached with greater caution by women who, due to the different profile of sex hormones, tend to react negatively to excessive calorie restriction and a sharp reduction in fat mass. In such cases, caution is required, and care should be taken not to reduce the calorie intake despite fasting excessively.

In some physiological periods, the practice of intermittent fasting is not recommended, as in pregnancy, nursing, childhood, and puberty. Nor is it appropriate in the event of an attempt to become pregnant.

Some special categories should avoid intermittent fasting if you suffer from:

-Hypoglycemia; Hypoglycaemia is the rapid lowering below normal blood sugar levels and represents the most frequent of the acute complications of diabetes. Hypoglycemia is more prevalent between meals and at night.

The causes may be non-compliance with diet schedule and type, unscheduled physical activity, insulin, or excessive oral hypoglycaemic intake.

-Diabetes; Diabetes is a chronic disease where there is an increase in blood sugar or blood sugar. This condition may be due to reduced insulin production, which has the task of transforming energy as assimilated by food or in other cases, the inability or reduced ability of the body to use insulin adequately. If high blood glucose levels are not corrected appropriately, complications of diabetes can become chronic, with damage to the heart and arteries, kidneys, and eyes as well as the peripheral nervous system. Coexisting with diabetes is not impossible, but it is essential to prevent complications resulting from the increase or decrease in blood sugar. Keeping it stable and within normal values is the necessary behavior to adopt, since the onset of the disease. And knowing what causes an increase or decrease in blood sugar in daily eating habits becomes crucial.

-Chronic stress; Stress consists of a state of dysfunction and alteration of the psych corporeal balance of the organism, which can become chronic and wear out the individual, for example, by losing the ability to develop responses and behaviors appropriate to real external needs. But stress is not necessarily a negative factor; on the contrary, if managed correctly, it can be a source of vitality and positive tension towards the achievement of one's fulfillment and well-being.

Once chronic, stress becomes highly harmful, as it forces the body into a situation of constant tension and alarms even when it would not be necessary, damaging its energy and health. It is now a fact that stress produces changes in all organs, through the mediation of the vegetative nervous system, the endocrine system, and the immune system, through a complex set of adjustment mechanisms.

-Imbalance of the cortisol; Cortisol is also called the stress hormone, as the body produces it under stress conditions, recognized by the body as a homeostasis disorder (cell balance with the environment). The body considers any event that can disrupt cellular or organic homeostasis as a stressing agent. The over-production of cortisol creates at first a "toxic" effect because the hormone counteracts the operation of brain cells deputed to a good mood, destroying them. In a second phase, however, when a natural mechanism of self-protection from cortisol occurs in the brain, if it is suddenly drastically reduced, it would create a cortisol deficiency in the brain cells, with consequent psychological and memory problems.

If you have a history of eating disorders, intermittent fasting is not recommended. People who are very underweight or who are currently fighting bulimia or anorexia should avoid IF or talk to their doctor first.

Hunger and adaptation to a new routine will be the main side effects of an IF protocol. In the early steps, you may experience some 'of mental fatigue or frustration, but it should disappear while you get used to the new routine.

Disorders such as:

-Sleep disorders (especially insomnia);

-disorders of the menstrual cycle (also during the intake of oral contraceptives);

-Increased irritability and/or anxiety;

-Physical and mental fatigue;

-A tendency to overeat or binge following a day

or a period of fasting;

-Chronic increase in hunger, especially for salty foods;

-Decrease of libido;

-Dry mouth and/or eyes;

-Symptoms are suggesting cortisol and/or blood glucose imbalance.

If affected, you should stop immediately and consult a doctor.

Conclusion

If you have decided to try intermittent fasting, keep in mind three general tips:

Remember that the quantity and quality of the food we eat are significant for health. The intermittent fasting should not be alternating with an incorrect diet.It is essential to record your emotional and physical state during fasting, to determine when it is necessary to suspend it. In this way, it also improves the level of awareness about the effects that food can have on the body and mind, a fundamental aspect of a healthy diet.

If you want to do a job on your body of quality, you can't ignore the physical exercise; this also probably implies a change in lifestyle, the real key to the success, and long-term maintenance of the results obtained.

In the beginning, it will be hard. Still, our organism has a strong capacity of adaptation, and, after the first days, with much probability, the continuation will be much less dramatic. Even cognitive abilities, mood, quality of sleep, and activity, in general, are not as strongly affected by fasting as one tends to believe. All this proves that the key to reading the initial malaise lies in the habit. So, either for the desperate quest to get positive effects for the last-minute costume fitting or because you had trouble staying true to other diets, if there are no particular individual problems, Intermittent fasting is also an option.

So intermittent fasting is a strategy to lose weight quickly and easily. The benefits that this diet provides are numerous, from improving physical fitness to longevity. However, this diet is not for everyone. You have to evaluate your health and avoid this diet if you are suffering from certain chronic diseases.

Among the VIPs who tested the intermittent fasting 16:8, there is also Jennifer Aniston. Jennifer, who usually gets up at 9:00 in the morning, begins her day with a juice of celery followed by an intensive session in the gym and, later, meditation.

Most of the information in this book has been selectively selected and compared. We used the web to document and deepen various scientific aspects (especially as regards research and experimental studies carried out over the years in the health and food sector), including the INRAN website, which has, for years, published scientific articles related to food. The texts have all been modified and adapted to the context.

It is essential to point out that after reaching the desired weight, you need to stop and adopt a healthy diet. The main goal of every diet to lose weight is also to maintain a healthy and active lifestyle even when you have reached the desired weight, Not To risk to accumulate fat again. We reiterate once again the importance of considering this book as a collection of information that should not replace the advice of a doctor. The choices they make every day will affect our future. In the case of food, for example, good manners begin at the table. Education should be taught from childhood to ward off a wrong approach to eating.

Thank you for purchasing the book.

We hope that the book was to your liking and as exhaustive as possible. The field of nutrition and nutrition-related to biology and how the whole affects the organism are extensive areas.

We also hope that you have understood the basic principles of intermittent fasting 16:8, how it works, what is preferable to eat, what hormones it affects, and how it works, its pros and cons.

Final Words

Thank you again for purchasing this book!

We hope this book can help you.

The next step is for you to join our email newsletter to receive updates on any upcoming new book releases or promotions. You can sign-up for free, and as a bonus, you will also receive our "*7 Fitness Mistakes You Don't Know You're Making*" book! This bonus book breaks down many of the most common fitness mistakes and will demystify many of the complexities and science of getting into shape. Having all this fitness knowledge and science organized into an actionable step-by-step book will help you get started in the right direction in your fitness journey! To join our free email newsletter and grab your free book, please visit the link and signup: www.effingopublishing.com/gift

Finally, if you enjoyed this book, then we would like to ask you for a favor, would you be kind enough to leave a review for this book? It would be much appreciated! Thank you, and good luck on your journey!

ABOUT THE CO-AUTHOR

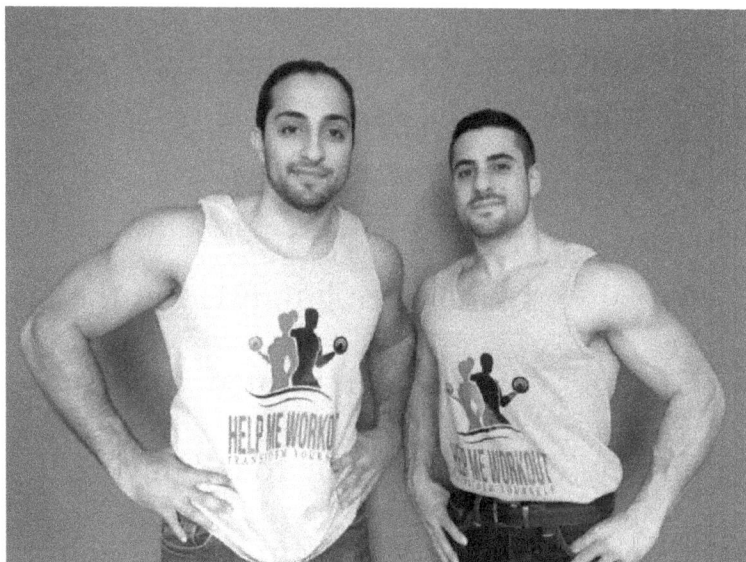

Our name is Alex & George Kaplo; we're both certified personal trainers from Montreal, Canada. We will start by saying we are not the biggest guys you will ever meet, and this has never really been our goal. We started working out to overcome our biggest insecurity when we were younger, which was our self-confidence. You may be going through some challenges right now, or you may want to get fit, and we can certainly relate.

We always kind were interested in the health & fitness world and wanted to gain some muscle due to the numerous bullying in our teenage years. We figured we could do something about how our body looks like. This was the beginning of our transformation journey. We had no idea where to start, but we both just got started. We felt worried and afraid at times that other people would make fun of us for doing the exercises the wrong way. We always wished we had a friend to guide us and who could show us the ropes.

After a lot of work, studying, and countless trials and errors. Some people began to notice how we were both getting more fit and how we were starting to form a keen interest in the topic. This led many friends and new faces to come to us and ask us for fitness advice. At first, it seemed odd when people asked us to help them get in shape. But what kept us going is when they started to see changes in their own body and told us it's the first time that they saw real results! From there, more people kept coming to us, and it made both of us realize after so much reading and studying in this field that it did help us, but it also allowed us to help others. To date, we have coached and trained numerous clients who have achieved some pretty amazing results.

Today, both of us own & operate this publishing business, where we bring passionate and expert authors to write about health and fitness topics. We also run an online fitness business, and we would love to connect with you by inviting you to visit the website on the following page and signing up for our e-mail newsletter (you will even get a free book).

Last but not least, if you are in the position we were once in and you want some guidance, don't hesitate and ask--I will be there to help you out!

Your coaches,

Alex &George Kaplo

Download another book for Free

We want to thank you for purchasing this book and offer you another book (just as long and valuable as this book), "Health & Fitness Mistakes You Don't Know You're Making," completely free.

Visit the link below to signup and receive it:

www.effingopublishing.com/gift

In this book, we will break down the most common health & fitness mistakes, you are probably committing right now, and will reveal how you can quickly get in the best shape of your life!

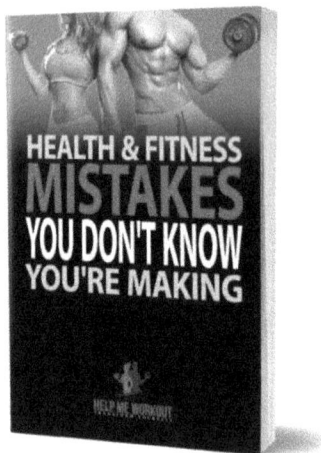

In addition to this valuable gift, you will also have an opportunity to get our new books for free, enter giveaways, and receive other useful emails from us. Again, visit the link to sign up:

www.effingopublishing.com/gift

The trademarks that are used are without any consent, and the publication of the trademark is without permission or backing by the trademark owner. All trademarks and brands within this book are for clarifying purposes only and are owned by the owners themselves, not affiliated with this document.

EFFINGO

Publishing

For more great books, visit:

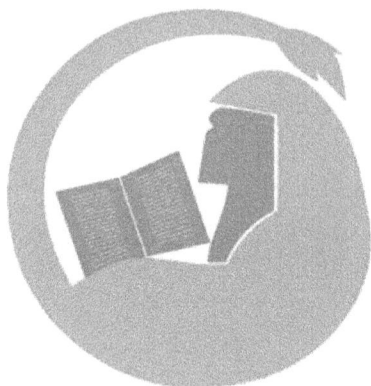

EffingoPublishing.com